Overview

Publishing is a very evasive art as it is in the modern day. So many different companies offer so many different plans, styles, printing methods, and sales methods that it is hard to know which publishing method to choose, let alone which company. Most websites offering information about publishing are advertisements for a publishing company or method. Advertisements can be untruthful and decidedly skirting around the point, leaving gaps in your knowledge and incorrect information in its place. This can make searching for the right method or company very difficult because you never know what wasn't told to you or what isn't true out of the stuff that was. However, the method I chose to publish this book is the method I consider to be best for the average person, with little or no financial risk and speedy printing and formatting. This method is most commonly referred to as "Print on Demand Publishing".

Print on Demand Publishing is a combination of Traditional Publishing and Self Publishing. Self Publishing is basically paying a company to print copies of your book, with each "package", or amount, of books costing a different amount of money. The Self Publishing company takes no percentage of the money made from sales, but also does not pay for advertising, or if they do they charge you extra because you went through their company to do it.

Traditional Publishing is the method that most people think of when they hear 'publishing'. It involves submitting a manuscript to a Publishing Agent, who is someone that will represent your book for you as you search for a company that will accept it to edit, format, advertise, and sell. These are the companies where they have a full staff of editors and salesmen to edit and sell books from various authors. They pay for advertising and editing, but a fairly large chunk of the profits go to the publishing company instead of your pocket.

Print on Demand Publishing, or "POD Publishing", is somewhat of an in-between of these two methods. It is a form of Self Publishing because your writing is accepted on the first try, no matter what the quality is. Necessities to publishing the book, like cover design, page layout, fonts, and pictures, are free at the point of use. However, once a copy of the book is purchased the writer must pay for the cost of printing and shipping, since Print on Demand Publishing means just that: a copy of the book is printed when there is a demand. The exact number of books printed is the number of books sold.

In order for this to work, the book doesn't actually exist when they buyer purchases it. Instead, the book is purchased off an online store such as Amazon. In this way, no money is wasted unless someone returns a book, so there is little or no financial risk in using this method and no waste is made. There is a downside to POD Publishing, though.

Although all necessary features of publishing are free at the point of use, extras like editing, advertising, and professional input on proofing, design suggestions, and marketing. Some different styles of books like hardcover, color printing, or different paper sizes may make the book cost more to print, but much of this still depends on the company.

The Differences Between Methods Step by Step

Self Publishing:

This is the most common method that comes to mind when people think about publishing a book themselves. In the simplest respect, Self Publishing is really just paying a printing company to print a number of copies of your writing. Although many different companies complete the formatting, editing, and printing of your book in different ways, this is the most common sequence of steps to Self Publish.

STEP 1: Write the book. Never consider doing this after you sign up for publishing. It is a lot easier to have the book ready and written by the time you visit the company's website and sign up for publishing.

STEP 2: Submit your writing to the company by signing up on the Self Publishing Company's website. Most websites give you options for formatting, cover design, page color and size, paperback or hardcover, color or black and white, et cetera, at this stage in the publishing process.

STEP 3: Pay the Self Publishing Company for a specific package of books that you wish to buy. The cost on these packages may vary depending on the number of books, number of pages in the books, and the colors presented in the book. If the book is in black and white it will probably be cheaper than if it is in color.

STEP 4: The Publishing Company reviews your book and makes minor changes if necessary to get it up to publishing standards. This can take a few days to a couple months depending on the length of the book and the availableness of the company.

STEP 5: You review your book to make sure it is the way you want it. If it is, you give the okay to the company and they print however many copies you ordered and ship them to you.

STEP 6: You figure out how to advertise and sell the bunches of copies you now have.

Traditional Publishing:

When people think 'publishing', this is the most common method that comes to mind and is the reason getting a book published seems so impossible. This is by far the method with the most steps, and, as an effect, takes the longest. However, if you are interested in really having your book out there and professionally edited, formatted, and advertised, if you don't mind the long tedious process, this is definitely the best method to publish a book in order to get business.

STEP 1: Write the book. If you don't do this first the rest of the steps cannot be completed, let alone successfully completed.

STEP 2: Submit your writing to a Publishing Agent. This is a person who will help advertise your book to publishing companies. They make your book look more professional and thus increase the chances of it getting published. This step can be skipped, but it is incredibly hard to get your book published traditionally, and when you don't have a Publishing Agent on your side it can be virtually impossible to get your book published.

STEP 3: Notice how step 2 only says to submit your writing to a Publishing Agent. That is because your writing is most likely to get rejected by the first Agent you submit it to. And the second, and the third, and who knows how many after that. That's why step 3 is to get rejected, because it is so unlikely to get accepted by a publishing agent on the first try that getting rejected has well earned a step of its own. Even if you skip this step by a magical stroke of luck, I can guarantee that this step will definitely happen later when you have to submit writing to the companies themselves.

STEP 4: Now that you have been rejected by countless Publishing Agents, it is about time you get accepted by one. It is advisable that you don't go on to step 5 if you don't complete this step. Publishing Agents don't just present your book to companies better, but they also help defend you when it comes to negotiating the percentage of profit that the company gets once the book is accepted and will help defend your case if the publishing company tries to take advantage of you.

STEP 5: Your Publishing Agent will now submit your writing to various Publishing Companies with a note explaining why they think your book is good enough to get published and why their company wants to jump on this chance to publish it. This step of 'bragging' about the book sounds a whole lot better when it is coming from someone that didn't write the book themselves, i.e., your Publishing Agent. Having a Publishing Agent also shows the company that you are serious about publishing your book, so they are more likely to consider it.

STEP 6: Fail and get rejected by the Publishing Companies many times. Often, the unpublished book will be returned to you by your Publishing Agent with an attached note saying why the company chose not to publish it. Sometimes, though, the book will simply be returned with a standard 'Thanks, but no thanks' letter from the Publishing Company. In some ways this is the most important step in Traditional Publishing, because without being rejected we would not know as much about what professional companies are looking for in terms of writing style, length, genre, plot line, character development, sentence structure, and so on. If you do decide to go with Traditional Publishing, it is definitely wise to read the notes and take account of them for future reference, or even change portions of your book before submitting it to a different company.

STEP 7: Finally, *finally* get accepted by a Publishing Company. There are many different variables that could account to the time it takes to get to this step in Traditional Publishing, so there is really no way to tell how long it will take. It could take anywhere from a couple months to a couple years, and most likely will take closer to the years end of the spectrum.

STEP 8: One of the Publishing Company's editors will be assigned to you, and he/she will edit the book on content, story plot, grammar, sentence structure, et cetera to get the book up to the publishing standard of the company. This editing process takes a very long time - most of the time years -, but can take more or less time depending on the quality and the length of the book. Obviously a short book is going to take less time than a long book to edit, but it also depends on how meticulous the editor or company is and the quality of the book before it has been edited.

STEP 9: After the editing process is done, the company will then proceed to making preliminary copies of the book to test formatting and binding. This step is not necessary and some companies may skip it. After this is done, you and/or a professional cover designer will decide on a cover design to put on the book's front and back.

STEP 10: When all of the final formatting decisions are made, final copies of the book will be printed, advertised, and sold by you and/or the company.

Print on Demand Publishing:

This is one of the least heard of out of the publishing methods. Not many people know what it is, how to use it, or even how to tell the difference between Print on Demand Publishing Companies and companies of other types. Print on Demand publishing is basically Self Publishing without any waste, since each copy of the book is only printed after a customer orders it. In this way there is little or no wasted paper or money and a very low financial risk, if any. In this way I believe Print on Demand Publishing is best for the average person. If you aren't really interested in selling a book and just really want to get your work published, this is definitely the best method. Even if you wrote the book to make money, most Print on Demand Publishing Companies offer advertising plans as well as editing and professional formatting plans.

STEP 1: Write the book. This is not the most necessary of steps in Print on Demand Publishing, but it is definitely recommended as a 'should', but it isn't exactly a definite 'must'.

STEP 2: Go on the publishing company's website and upload your writing to the page. Most companies will also give you an option to format it in this stage of publishing.

STEP 3: Complete the necessary items on the company's list of things to publish a book. Most non-necessary things and special things that are necessary will cost extra. Like editing, professional formatting, professional cover design, and so on.

STEP 4: Once all of these steps are completed, you submit it to the company, who views it and makes sure it is suitable and up to publishing standards. They might ask you to make a few changes.

STEP 5: Once the company gives the okay, you review it one last time to make sure you like it and that all of the formatting is correct. If you are okay with it, you submit it again and the Publishing Company prints and ships however many copies you ordered for yourself and then puts the book on their online purchasing website for other people to buy. You get to set the price, and once someone buys a copy you pay for the printing and get to keep the money left over from the sale. The only way you can lose money is if someone returns a book.

Pros and Cons of Each

Self Publishing:

Pros	Cons
- The Publishing Company gets no percentage of sales - Quick and easy way to get published - Any book gets published, no matter what the quality - Best if you are experienced in sales and think you can market and sell your book better by yourself	- You advertise and sell the books; there is no bookstore or website to help you - All of the money for printing comes out of your pocket, and much of that 'printing money' actually goes towards the company itself - You have to decide how many copies of your book you want that you think you will be able to sell right then and there

Traditional Publishing:

Pros	Cons
- Company advertises and sells for you; easier sales	- Very long and tedious process
- Professional editing, cover design, interior design, et cetera	- Hard to get companies to accept your book to publish it
- People who know what they are doing walk you through each step of publishing	- Publishing Company gets to take a percentage of the profits for themselves
- Best if you want a job as a writer	
- Helps get your name out there better than other methods	

Print on Demand Publishing:

Pros	Cons
- Quick and easy process	- Editing and other extras cost more
- Little waste, if any	- Formatting, editing, and cover design can be tricky if you want to do them yourselves so you don't have to pay for them
- Optional professional add-ons, like cover design, editing, and advertisement	
- Best for the average person	

Commonly Asked Questions

Q: Which publishing method is best?

A: As with anything, there is really no way to tell which method is the best one to use, because it all depends on the circumstances. If you are really good with sales and advertisement and think you would be better off selling your book yourself, you should definitely consider Self Publishing as a viable option. If you really love writing and want to create an off-the-charts best-seller, Traditional Publishing is probably best for you because all of the advertising and sales are done by the company. But if you are like me, and just want to see your work out there without really caring whether it sells well or not, then you should definitely choose Print on Demand publishing because of its speedy printing and formatting and because there is little or no financial risk involved

Q: Which method is the easiest?

A: Without a doubt, the easiest method to use is Print on Demand Publishing. With its easy-to-follow steps, speedy printing and formatting, abundant personalization options, and aversion to financial risk and waste, POD publishing is the publishing method for the average person.

Q: How long will it take?

A: There is no way to tell exactly how long it will take, as every book, editor, and company is different, but there is a range that your book should fall into depending on which method you choose to use to publish it. Traditional Publishing could take anywhere from a couple months to a few years, but most likely it will take at least a couple months just to find a Publishing Agent, so it is more likely to take years. Self Publishing, however, is really up to you. If you have everything written and perfected when you submit it to the company, then it will take hardly any time at all. If you decide you want to edit it professionally through the Self Publishing company you're using, then it will most likely take a few months. The same is true for Print on Demand publishing. However, whichever method you choose to use, the brunt of all the work is always in the writing of the book.

Acknowledgements

Almost all of the information in this book was either gathered from my personal experiences or from Harvey Chapman's webpage on precisely this topic. His webpage covers everything in this book plus a few extras, like how to publish an eBook and even some helpful hints on how to write novels, so if you are really interested in this topic you should definitely check it out at

www.novel-writing-help.com/publishing-a-novel.html

Also, if you're interested in using the Print on Demand publishing company I used, you can visit their website at

www.createspace.com

About the Author

I am currently fourteen years old and am in the eighth grade. This is the first book I have ever published, but I have two others that I am writing as of now. I live in California as I have all my life with my parents and my younger sister.

I have dreamt of becoming a published author all of my life and the pressure of having a report to do has finally given me a reason to accomplish this. I never thought I'd say this, but thank you Campbell Union School District for assigning me this incredibly long and involved report. No joke!

www.ingramcontent.com/pod-product-compliance
Lightning Source LLC
Chambersburg PA
CBHW060342290526

45793CB00003B/704